Release

YOUR INNER

BEAST

EMBRACE YOUR INNER
ENDO WARRIOR

CARLA RODRIGUES, DVM, CCRP, CVA

Thank you to every single person that has been part of my journey, in a positive way, past and present. You all know who you are. I am so fortunate to continuously have genuine and loyal support anywhere I go, and for that I will eternally be grateful.

Special thanks to ...

My parents:
You've always worked so hard for what you have; thank you for instilling this in me.

My sister Paula:
There is no one in life like a sister. Thank you for sharing so many memories and having such a big heart. Your kids are so lucky to have the super mom you are.

My Aunt Lurdes:
You have always truly been an inspiration. You are the reason for the initial spark to my fire and have never faltered when I've needed guidance and encouragement. You define strength and are a role model for any dedicated working mother.

Jackie:

Thank you for sharing your amazing energy and wisdom with me.

The ADCH Crew:

Anyone I have met through my connection with Arlington Dog & Cat Hospital. Your sincere support and friendships have and will always be a shining light in my life. Des, thanks for your continuous input and support.

My Rossies and Island Family:

I love you all.

Stella and Jackson:

My rescue mutts, my heart.

I am so grateful.

Stay connected:
www.awarriorwithinyou.com
www.endocenter.org

Thank you to everyone involved in making this book possible:

Cover and author photo by Sara Moynier
https://www.focusflash.co/
Cover design by Immaculate Studios
Editing by Katie Chambers http://beaconpointservices.org/
Proofreading by Danielle Decker http://deckerswordshop.com/
Formatting by Nerdy Wordsmith and Likhar Publishing

This is my own personal story. This book is not intended to give medical advice nor substitute for the medical advice of physicians. The reader should make medical decisions based on their own judgement and regularly consult a physician in matters relating to his/her health and particularly with respect to any symptoms that may require diagnosis or medical attention.

ISBN: 978-1-7342997-0-0

CONTENTS

PREFACE

*P*icture it: I was on my way to Malibu, California, at an intersection, just about to turn on to the Pacific Coast Highway, when a thought hit me like a lightning bolt: I should write a book.

I had just completed a self-tour of Los Angeles, mainly for old times' sake. When I lived in Southern California, the undeniable wanderlust within would take me to places like Joshua Tree National Park, San Diego, Los Angeles and Palm Springs. So it's no surprise the act of driving around with no exact destination rekindled fond memories of endless exploration and joy. It was a very reflective trip for me. While the purpose was to visit some very close and endearing friends in Southern California, I knew the days away would give me much needed quality time with myself.

My thoughts streamed, from one to another, with no interruption. Flashing back to my days in California and realizing that was a different time in my life, I found myself tracing my path from northern New Jersey, which I call my true home; to veterinary school in St. Kitts; to my clinical year at the University of Minnesota; to California, straight out of vet school; to Charlotte, North Carolina; and now Jacksonville, Florida. There is no doubt why I moved from one place to another. Aside from my interest in living in different places and my natural nomadic tendencies, the motive behind those moves was my longing for a well-balanced, fulfilling career.

After all, I had dedicated my life to my career. I left home; I left my family. I had a fire inside me that would not be extinguished until I felt like I had reached my goal of becoming a veterinarian. My mind then dove to a deeper place within the trenches of my subconscious to precisely where this fire had originally been ignited, fueled by my days of endometriosis and continuous struggle to find myself. This was a time when I was tested and pushed to my limits. It was a time of incredible growth and the very beginning of my journey to discovering self-worth and putting myself first. This journey is perpetual and continues on to this day. There are still times I sit and wonder where my endometriosis came from. Why did it flourish in my body? Was there something I could have done to avoid it? Although it's taken several years, I've come to terms that there are no answers to those questions, and there won't be. But this doesn't mean I can't do everything in my power to keep it away, forever. It also won't stop me from using my experience to help others who are in the same boat.

It would make sense if resentment remained my default response to these circumstances I had absolutely no say in — along with anger, frustration and fear. However, I've chosen to rise above this mysterious disease, and I'm sticking to that choice. Despite the struggle and pain that has been handed to me, I know now, more than ever, that I wouldn't be who I am today if it weren't for endometriosis. If you're wondering if this means that I'm okay that this happened to me, the answer is yes and no. Because my evolution in the last 15 years has been so closely interlaced with the obstacles I faced with endometriosis and associated conditions, I can argue that I'm grateful for the person it has made me today. I truly believe everything happens for a reason, and that has comforted me through the years, especially as I've watched my life unravel right before my eyes, year after year. I sincerely trust that now is the right time to share my story.

So, welcome to my story. That day on my way to Malibu, I decided I'd put it all down on paper, with the hope that I would reach out to as many people as possible. My heartfelt intention in writing this book is not just for endometriosis victims, but for anyone feeling like they're fighting an uphill battle and need reassurance that they're not alone. Despite there being over 175 million women affected by endometriosis in this world and millions of other men and women struggling through countless health or mental health issues, those diagnosed still feel a lingering disconnect and deep loneliness. As human beings, we share a need for connecting with others and for knowing that we're not the only ones feeling what we're feeling. It's critical to be encouraged by others' triumphs or victories. This is because we then know it is possible! It can be done.

Please understand this book is not intended to serve as medical advice or imply that every single person's journey is the same and destined to have the same ending. Nor am I discrediting any doctors' hard work and practice or pharmaceutical companies, by any means. This is not my intent.

My book is here as a reflection of my own path from diagnosis to where I am now; however, this may help you in your own unique journey. I genuinely hope that reading this book will resonate with you on some level and bring encouragement to you or others around you. Whether my words inspire you to take full action and make life-changing choices or simply put a smile on your face, I have succeeded.

Whatever your story or your intention for picking up this book may be, I hope you find a sense of commonality and realize you're not alone. Hopefully, you'll see life in a different light. Whether you've been diagnosed specifically with endometriosis or another chronic condition, you know someone going through a difficult time medically or in life, or you're looking for some overall encouragement and need a boost of confidence, you've come to the right place. There's a peaceful reassurance that comes with knowing we're not facing something alone. Sharing our stories and experiences can make a tremendous impact on others' lives, not to mention give hope. Everyone has a story. Don't be afraid to own yours and share it.

Regardless of our stories, we all work toward finding balance and harmony.

For most, balance and harmony are only a dream. They're some kind of far away, unreachable fantasy-world undertaking that can only be realized in a fictional world or only very selectively granted to special divine people chosen by the heavens above. Must be nice, people say to me all the time. I cringe every time. If you haven't already, once your warrior helps you achieve a harmonious state, don't succumb to the "must be nices." Stand up for yourself. Make it known to those haters that you're in a state of balance and harmony because you worked your ass off to get there! You made it a priority, now this is your prerogative. They, too, can achieve bliss, find self-love, repel stress, cleanse themselves of toxic people and be the best versions of themselves if they want to! It all starts with desire.

I'm here to tell you it is all possible. All you need is some guidance, discipline, this book, and a really, really, really strong desire to be pain free and live happily ever after.

Is that too much to ask for? It's unbelievable to me that true health and balance tend to be the exception to the rule. Disappointment is the word that comes to mind when I think about how many times (not always) true balance takes priority only after our well-being is at risk. Only then do we realize how good we had it before our diagnosis and how much we've taken our health for granted.

Please join me in raising awareness for endometriosis and any other dreadful conditions, especially those that are taking the lives of so many loved ones. Find the courage within yourself to really focus on who you are and what you want out of your own life. Be your own voice; be the voice for others. Find the support you need and keep focused. Be an inspiration. Don't ever forget that you, and only you, hold the key to your own health and happiness. Be the creator of your own narrative and watch the magic happen. Your inner beast will thank you.

Love yourself.

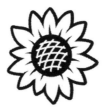

Part One: My Story

FORGET FEAR

We hear it over and over again — life is hard. Three words that are so meaningful, yet so vague. Who came up with this brief but powerful quote, anyway? There's no one to claim it; however, it resonates within almost every being on this earth. While there is an undeniable truth to those words, wouldn't it be so much better if we walked around saying life is what you make of it?

We, and only we, have the power to define ourselves and our lives. We, and only we, have the power to make our own decisions and mold our lives into what we want them to be. As humans, our intricate and complex minds have so much to face with external stimuli awaiting us every day as we trudge through our busy lives. The mind is a beautiful thing; the mind is also a very profoundly and deeply daunting thing, so easily persuaded and swayed by continuous messages from the outside world.

With the immense growth of social media in the last 15 years, it's no shock to see insecurity, judgment, jealousy and lack of confidence — just to name a few — rear their ugly heads, while people's identities slowly fizzle away and their sense of self becomes consigned to the oblivion of the "other." Hey "other," what did you do to sense of "self"?

Social acceptance is so intricately woven into our existence, it sneaks into our psyche without notice. What is your first knee-jerk reaction when you're faced with an important decision? Do you think, how will this be perceived by others? What if I don't make the right decision? Ladies and gentlemen, meet fear. The four-letter word that has kept, and will continue to keep millions of people from their sincere happiness. Fear so skillfully keeps our thoughts in captivity, like the weight of a ball and chain preventing us from moving forward.

Now, if fear, insecurity and the rest of the negative bandits are a given in our existence, this leads us to wonder what happens when we face hurdles and feel like we can't quite clear the rim? That already weakened self collapses, time after time. We're forced to build back up, even when the proper building blocks were not there to begin with.

With each experience we face, we add another building block to our foundation. These building blocks are discovered one by one, each time we reach to clear a hurdle. On the other side of those hurdles is reassurance. It's human nature to crave reassurance as we triumph over upward challenges simply because we then know what is possible and all doubt is removed. No doubt, no worry — more confidence. The more you fall and get right back up, the less you hesitate to clear each hurdle. It may be a difficult race, but boy is it worth it in the end.

Besides, what are these building blocks I speak of? The crucial building blocks vital to resilience are your trustworthy friends called confidence, integrity, determination, strength, hope, courage, self-love and my favorite — warrior. Dig deep because I promise you, these guys are within you. They just need some discovery and inspiration.

WHEN LIFE HANDS YOU LEMONS

I've been called unconventional many times. It's not a bad word, although I prefer individualistic; nonetheless, I feel like it can be a character-defining word. Do you agree?

Regardless of its interpretation, to me, it represents everything I stand for. With individualism comes self. It's difficult to think that it's so much easier to hang with the ugly bandits than to discover our sense of self. Why do we need to find our "self" anyway?! Why isn't it just right there, prepped and ready to go conquer the world?! Well, that would be too easy.

I was a typical 20-year-old, minding my own business, attending college at Montclair State University in my home state of New Jersey as a full-time biology student, with a minor in English literature. Biology came naturally to me. I am a scientist at heart. The inner workings and mechanisms of a living organism will never cease to amaze me. After a couple of years of not choosing a major, I finally decided I needed to stop being in denial about what my heart was telling me to do. My calling? Veterinary medicine. My love of animals has always been there. However, my connection with animals on a deeper level became very apparent during my time working as a veterinary assistant at Arlington Dog & Cat Hospital in my hometown. I spent eight years of my life working alongside veterinarians and technicians that took me under their wings and became my second family. ADCH was so much a part of my existence. It's a good thing because my job ultimately became my escape.

One night in March 2004, I suddenly felt a very sharp pain in my abdomen. Sharp doesn't even describe the agony of this pain. It was very specific in location and didn't budge. While I was hoping the first few stabs of pain were just temporary and would go away, it didn't take me long to figure out they weren't going anywhere, and I found myself struggling to stand. This moment was the beginning of a long road to recovery and discovery. I just didn't quite know it yet.

Never a dull moment

I naturally went downstairs as gracefully as one could when doubled over in pain. My mother caught sight of me and did what any concerned mother would do: took me to the hospital. What a blur. To think that was the first visit of many in the upcoming year! They appropriately called for an MRI to assess what was going on inside of me. They were concerned about appendicitis. Before I knew it, I was all hooked up to all sorts of lines, lying there wondering what just happened. Anxiety. Fear. My mind was racing; what will happen next? Okay, I'm sure the drugs and painkillers they had me on to suppress the pain may have had a little to do with the mind racing and confusion, but I wouldn't give them all the credit. Anxiety and fear just jumped on the bandwagon and went for a ride.

When the results came in, I wasn't sure whether to be relieved or even more concerned. I had fluid present in my abdomen as a result of a ruptured ovarian cyst. Oh, ovary!

Ovaries seem to get forgotten and are obviously subordinate to the mighty appendix. The good — that meant no emergency appendectomy. The bad — but what did it mean? The doctor assured me that with some pain medications and rest, I would recover and move on with my life. If that were the case, this would be the end of my story.

I was referred to my general gynecologist for the continuation of care and management of my condition. Once again, a ruptured ovarian cyst is no biggie, they say. After all, cysts (a.k.a. follicular cysts) are part of every woman's reproductive function. Month to month, the egg that is ready to be released out into the open range of your uterus is housed within a follicle. If the follicle fails to rupture to release the egg as per the rules, fluid accumulates, and therefore a follicular cyst is born. Now, the egg can make it out of the follicle as expected, and a cyst can still make itself known — this one is called a corpus luteum cyst.

By definition, any cyst is a fluid-filled sac. So, here we are with a fluid-filled bubble that has the potential to keep growing, sitting on our ovary. It has no purpose other than to sit there, cause pain, release hormones and maybe decide to resolve on its own. Or maybe not.

Recheck after recheck after recheck, my gynecologist assured me that the cyst had resolved along with the fluid in my abdomen. Then why, I asked time after time, do I still feel pain? The doctor at the time expressed his concern for a condition called endometriosis. Everything around me froze in time a little bit. Endometriosis sounds like a disease. Oh, it is a disease. Glad I got clarity on that.

He explained the only way to know whether endometriosis was a factor in my continuous discomfort was to go in by laparoscopy and biopsy abnormal tissue for confirmation. I walked out of the office in a daze. Here came fear, and here came anxiety. That fear and anxiety stuck around for a while.

The researcher in me went straight to the internet to see what endometriosis was all about, and I didn't like what I was reading. So I did what any other fearful human being would do: I tried to ignore it and allowed denial to move right in and join its long-time friends, anxiety and fear. Besides, the pain didn't happen all the time; it was on and off. Maybe it was all in my head, I kept telling myself. Every time I was ready to make a move toward diagnosis, the pain would go away and I would succumb to the deceiving denial again. This vicious cycle continued for a few months before I decided I needed to know. It took four months, to be exact. In August 2004, I went in for my biopsy.

The results would change my life forever.

BABY WARRIOR

*W*hat to do, what to do. Regardless of the words written on paper, my mind relentlessly clung on to denial. Maybe if I didn't think about it, it would go away. Realistically, I knew this wouldn't be the case. By this time, I had done much more research on endometriosis. It was surely a thing, a thing that was in my body and ready to wreak havoc. Because the information I was reading didn't settle well with me, I went from resource to resource hoping one of them would say something different. They were all the same, page after page! Why can't someone tell me something different?! "Carla," denial would whisper, "keep looking. Don't believe everything you read." Denial was a sneaky, misleading little bugger. It didn't take too long before frustration and anger joined the party, too.

Someone please tell me why there is endometrial-like tissue causing pain inside me. How on earth did it decide to appear on my organs? The disease process of endometriosis is most commonly described as the atypical existence of endometrial-like tissue within the abdominal cavity, on extrauterine sites. Back in my day, my research consisted of resources labeling endometrial lesions as pieces of endometrial tissue that possibly retrograded out of the uterus and found themselves lost within my abdomen. This concept was much more accepted at that time. Researchers are not as supportive of this theory today. The truth is, we don't know. No researcher has found a definitive answer. We need to know more. This is why it is imperative we start recognizing the scope of the complexity of endometriosis and its debilitating effects. It's not just a big deal, it's a major deal.

Not everyone experiences the same degree of pain, and there have been many different ways women have described their endometriosis pain. I personally equated my crippling pain to pouring liquid acid into my abdomen, all the time. Endometriosis can be classified into one of four stages: Stage 1, being mild, to Stage 4, the most severe. The general classification is based on location, the number of lesions, depth, size and the extent of spread of endometrial lesions. While the implants most commonly stick to the ovaries themselves, they can very easily go anywhere they damn please. The bladder, colon, pelvic wall, upper intestinal tract, the kidneys, you name it — all are at risk of an unexpected visitor. At this time, I was not aware of my stage quite yet. We can call it my baby warrior stage.

YOU ARE NOT ALONE

*T*here are five stages to the process of grief. Grief is the response to loss. Conventionally, we relate grief specifically to the loss of a loved one or family member. Anyone that has been through this agonizing process knows what a helpless time it can be. We may all be different when it comes to our individuality, beliefs and existence as a people on this earth, but no one can deny some of the common bonds we all have as human beings. One of them is the process of grief or loss. No matter what color, what culture, what religion you follow or what ethnicity you are, there is no escaping the grasp of grief. Some may think they handle it well on the outside, but you can only hide it so long on the inside.

Benjamin Franklin had once written that nothing in this world can be said to be certain except death and taxes. Such a wise man he was. So true a statement that illustrates everyone will experience loss at one time or another in their lives. Unfortunately, most will experience grief more than once, time after time. Although losing a loved one is by far the most potent form of grief anyone can experience, grief can make itself known in other situations. Ever lost your job? Lost a friendship? Lost your pet? Gotten a divorce? Had to move away from a place you loved? Lost trust in somebody? You may not have been aware, but grief was right there alongside you as you navigated yourself to the next step. Just because grief has five distinct stages, this doesn't mean the duration of each stage needs to be the same each and every time. It is unique to every situation and everyone.

In the case of facing a medical diagnosis or condition, we have a sense of loss for our previous selves. The loss of the person we were up until someone labeled us with a disease that we now have no choice but to bear.

When my anger and frustration set in, I had reached stage two of the grief process. Of course, I didn't know this at the time. I was just naturally going through the motions. The never-ending why's, what's and how's made their appearance.

Why is this happening now?

Why didn't I have any symptoms before?

What did I do to cause this?

What can I do?

Why is it so painful?

Why did this cyst have to develop?

What is my next step?

How do I tell people?

How will people respond?

What does this mean for my education and career?

Just why?

The one obvious person to turn to was my doctor. As grateful as I was that my gynecologist recognized the red flags pretty readily and succeeded in identifying my mysterious chronic pain, I still felt empty with so many unanswered questions. It was mind-blowing to learn how common it was for women to go undiagnosed for years! Years! How was this possible? How are we allowing women to experience this kind of pain unnoticed? I repeatedly reminded myself to be grateful for at least knowing what I was up against. Now to figure out how to defeat it.

SAYS WHO?

At this stage, I was still very vulnerable, lost and confused. I wondered what I had done to cause this. I read books and articles and joined online forums to no avail. Everyone seemed to be in the same boat as I. Hundreds of women online expressed their helpless coexistence with chronic debilitating pain.

My first visit back to my gynecologist after I received my diagnosis was not as liberating as I hoped it would be. I envisioned walking out of the office with a clear plan and optimism for my future without endometriosis. Even though I had read a thousand times that there is no cure for endometriosis, I was in denial. Besides, maybe they had found a cure overnight.

My doctor indeed reiterated what I had read time after time: there is no cure. At the time, the only options he discussed with me involved hormone treatments aimed to minimize the severity of pain and prevent further development of implants. Being a baby warrior in denial, I accepted this fate and asked what the next step was for hormone treatment. Since the lesions respond to hormones just as the endometrium does during a normal menstrual cycle (they theorized at the time), it would only make sense to minimize the amount of estrogen stimulation available to the detrimental implants. This hormone injection contained the synthetic hormone progestin, and I would need to get it every three months. The idea was to create a state of chemical menopause — no ovulation, no monthly bleeding. Sounded simple and straightforward. A small bit of me still wanted more. What if I tried other things, like focusing on nutrition and being very good about what I put inside my body? What if I just gave it more time before committing to these injections? I introduced denial and bargaining as accomplices. This phase didn't last too long, mainly because depression was right around the corner waiting its turn.

INNER BEAST — PLEASE STAND UP

*L*ooking back, I realize I experienced a combination of every emotion possible, at any given time. While denial and anger still stuck around, depression had no qualms about joining the group and making itself comfortable. I was in a vulnerable state. Hormone treatment had begun and a plan had been laid out, yet it was all still so unclear and foggy to me. The doctor had warned me that hormone treatment would possibly have an effect on my disposition, with mood swings being the most common possibility. Although the word menopause had been introduced during the discussion, I hadn't stopped to really think about the full implication of that. I never thought I would know the true meaning of hot flashes at the age of 21. They were more like fire flashes! The sudden rise of heat in my face, accompanied by a patchy pattern of flushed skin all over my body, led me to duck into restrooms more often than I could count.

There's no better way to put it: I was a walking time bomb. I remember thinking, how on earth do I not have any control over what I'm doing? It's true. My typical Jersey road rage multiplied by 10. I had absolutely no tolerance or patience for anyone; it didn't matter what they had to say. The daily pressures of everyday life were getting to me. I didn't want to talk to anyone. I spent my time at home in my bedroom, on my bed, doubled over in pain, wondering day after day what would come of my life if this continued this way. My heating pad became my friend; I always had it within reach. I cried. I cried a lot. As easily as anger set in, so did sadness and the helpless feeling of not knowing what to do next.

Ultimately, as my condition worsened, I was faced with a very difficult decision. I was a full-time student at Montclair State, and each day was an upward battle. The difficulty of physically getting to class, sitting in class and being expected to focus became too much for me. My Type A personality did not appreciate this. It was one of the most difficult decisions I had to make, but I reluctantly decided to take a semester off school so I could have time to recover and get back on my feet. I knew it was the right thing to do at that time, but it didn't mean I was happy about it. However, despite my hiatus from school, the stubborn mule in me would not stop working. My part-time position as a veterinary assistant became part of my coping mechanism. Joining my colleagues almost every day in helping animals and people alike gave me some relief mentally, if not physically. I'll admit, being on my feet and working with animals was not exactly what the doctor ordered, but I was willing to endure the pain. That's how much that job meant to me. It was either be in pain at work while doing what I loved, or be in pain at home, on my bed, staring at the ceiling, crying.

The crew at Arlington Dog & Cat Hospital, to this day, remain a second family to me. The amount of support and encouragement I felt in their presence was enough to help me forget my body was being invaded by a disease process, even for a split second. Day after day, I went to work, did what I needed to do and went back to my solitary bed.

After several months of this mundane cycle, I decided I would ask my doctor if there was another option we could consider. I had received several hormone injections and truly felt like there was no change for the better. Every day was a challenge. The endo pain itself was no longer localized to one area and resonated higher into my abdomen, down to my lower back. To add fuel to the fire, the injection itself would cause additional discomfort. I could barely stand on my leg some days. I had acquired a limp that changed my gait. This was my way of adjusting and compensating for the stubborn pain that had taken over the right side of my lower body.

Here I was, almost 22 by now, feeling pretty close to defeated. As time passed, I took semester after semester off, with no resolution to my aching pain. If my world wasn't upside down already, the next option I asked the doctor about was about to flip it.

In short, the next several months were worse than the last. My gynecologist turned to the other commonly used hormone treatment: a gonadotropin-releasing hormone agonist (GnRHa). A mouthful that means we wanted to suppress the amount of estrogen stimulation in my body again. Except this time, we would ask my pituitary gland to stop sending signals for estrogen. I was told it was the only other option for my endometriosis pain, and it was a monthly injection. My naïve, desperate self signed up for the treatment. My future educated warrior self looks back and wants to hit my doctor over the head with my shoe! In the course of the next six months, I experienced the following:

- Severe weakness and dullness
- Neutropenia (abnormally low number of neutrophils, a white blood cell)
- Walking pneumonia that lasted over six months
- Several hospitalizations
- A bone biopsy to investigate the neutropenia
- Fainting spells
- Being rejected as a blood donor (I was not healthy enough)

The new hormone treatment made a dent all right. During those six months, the most difficult part for me to accept was that I learned my latest hormone treatment was considered a chemotherapy drug. I only learned of this when I was rejected at a blood drive. I wanted to donate blood for a sick friend undergoing cancer. Imagine my surprise when, during the screening process, they informed me that I didn't qualify to donate due to being on chemotherapy. My world crumbled. Now it all made sense. The neutropenia led to my pneumonia. I had no immune defenses.

Continuously feeling like I had no energy, I sat down any chance I got. It all became clear. I cried, and

I cried, and I cried. I felt so violated. My body was made to be an experiment with a drug that did me much more harm than good. I was never informed of the extent of the impact this drug could have on my body — not just at that time, but long term.

Sprinkled among my eclectic group of doctors and specialists was now a rheumatologist. I had been referred to him because I was experiencing nonstop joint and muscle pain. I was still so weak, and I had continuous muscle twitches. My mind was foggy, and my body felt heavy. It was difficult for me to get up in the mornings, and I felt like my gas tank was empty all the time.

It was at the rheumatologist's office that I learned of the irreversible damage the hormone treatment may have done to my body. He ran extensive tests, even checking me for Lyme disease — the whole gamut. His diagnosis of exclusion was fibromyalgia. Wonderful. Here we go again.

My fingers pounded the keys looking for information on fibromyalgia. It was indeed listed as a possible side effect of the drug. Every site I read defined fibro more or less as a widespread musculoskeletal disorder with a wide range of symptoms, treatment and management options. Mainly, it's characterized by muscular pain and stiffness with very heavy fatigue that lingers and lingers and lingers. Well, that sounded about right.

I was hormonal, I was in pain and I was close to giving up. Until I decided I wouldn't stand for it. Once I got the emotions out of the way, I knew I could not keep living my life like this. I had reached my breaking point. I thought of my education, my dream of becoming a veterinarian and my desire to have children. All this down the drain because my doctor had no more options for me? I realized my happiness was in question. I was not about to settle for a shrug.

My next visit to my gynecologist would be my last. I expressed my concern and asked one more time for any other options. He looked me straight in the eyes and told me he would write me a prescription for Vicodin and that I would just have to live with it. Just have to live with it … those words still ring in my ears as vibrant as they were that day.

That is when my inner beast first came out to play.

DON'T BE SHY

*I*t's kind of unfair sometimes how we seem to feel like it's necessary to sustain a certain amount of hardships before we finally decide it's time to rise up. It just kind of happens as human beings, or at least it did for me. I know people out there that start conquering right from the beginning. The majority, however, can't help but go through the motions of emotions, the grief and the depression, before we stand up for our own rights as advocates for our own health. It should be the norm to spring into action from the moment there is any suspicion or concern. Instead, we have all these pre-set doubts and roadblocks that really don't have any valid foundation for existence. None. It's fear. If you're asking why, the answer is fear.

What are people going to think?

What if I'm wrong?

What if it's all in my head?

What if people don't believe me?

What if I find no one that will listen or care?

Who am I to say anything?

What gives me the right to challenge others?

Do I have what it takes to see it all the way through?

Would it just be easier to deal with it?

Here are the answers:

What are people going to think?

They won't think anything. They will only think they want to help or maybe find someone that can help you. They will also admire your courage.

What if I'm wrong?

You're not. And let's say with the slightest chance you are, who cares?!

What if it's all in my head?

It's not.

What if people don't believe me?

Keep looking until they do. Find the right people and resources.

What if I find no one that will listen or care?

You will. Plenty of people are committed to the cause and in the same boat.

Who am I to say anything?

You are you and deserve every bit of help and attention as anyone else does. Believe in yourself and be true to yourself.

What gives me the right to challenge others?

Your right to live your life happily and endo free.

Do I have what it takes to see it all the way through?

No doubt. This is what this book is all about. You've already started with step one.

Would it just be easier to deal with it?

Gasp. No. Sure, it may be easier to succumb and mundanely continue living your life, but are you really happy with this? You have the power within you.

Why can't I just do nothing?

*Why can't you just do **something**?*

There's no doubt what the elephant in the room is — many women are too embarrassed or shy to address endometriosis specifically because it has to do with the female reproductive system. For many, this can be a delicate and sensitive subject to talk about. It's personal, very personal. Who wants to talk to doctors about their uterus, their sex lives, their menstrual cycles? No one. But realize it's not just you. This is very important to understand. You're not the only one going through these changes, and no one will judge you for them. You and every other one of the 174,999,999 women in the world that are affected by endometriosis are going through this at the same time. The only difference is you may be in a different state, country or even continent from the others. Please understand, everything you're feeling, doubting, confused about, uncertain of, scared of, questioning, worried about — you name it — is absolutely acceptable for what you are going through.

EMPOWER YOURSELF

*A*nger, frustration, fear, anxiety, guilt, regret. Did I say anger? I was outraged at my situation. A year of my life had gone by with no improvement. In fact, I was worse. By this time, I could feel the endo pain spreading even more. How could I have allowed this to happen? Why didn't I look into the treatment options further? Because I was scared and I needed someone to hold my hand, that's why. If this sounds like you at times, there's nothing wrong with you. Trust me.

My quest to find answers began. I must have seen at least 10 other gynecologists for second, third, fourth and fifth opinions … they all had the same thing to say. It was like listening to a broken record. Not one of them could give me a different answer: there is no cure. Too bad, I'm not taking this as an answer anymore. I researched, researched and researched until I came across an endometriosis specialty surgeon who offered surgical endometriosis excision. Apparently, they were hard to come by, and there were only a few in the United States at the time. This one was located in Atlanta, Georgia. He could have been located in Timbuktu; I was set on going.

With this newfound fury and determination, I continued to research. The more I delved into the endo world, the more treasure I uncovered. The biggest jewel of them all? Finding out surgical excision was an option.

Up until now, not one person had mentioned this to me. I had seen more than 10 gynecologists looking incredulously for options, and no one thought to mention surgery as an option. It was flabbergasting. Just tell me! Let me make the decision whether I'd like to pursue that route or not. It's my body and my uterus. Is it because they felt like they would be opening up a can of worms if they mentioned it? Maybe they didn't believe it would be successful. Inform your patients. Let them decide. It's my can, and it's my worms.

Once I realized an actual surgery existed, I felt like I was given a divine key to a door that few people knew existed. Never mind the fact that the first and only surgeon I had come across, at that time, was located several states away. Minor detail. I skipped right over the location and started reading the procedure, prognosis, expectations, recovery and consultation options.

I picked up the phone and shook as I dialed the number. As my conversation with the office coordinator progressed, I could feel a body-wide sensation, a wave of emotion zipping through my chest. I felt my pulse in my throat. Thoughts raced through my mind as I tried to keep myself calm so I could absorb everything she was saying to me. "Our success rate is very high with endometriosis excision," she advised me. Excision. Hmm. I welcomed anything with the word *ex* in it when it came to endo. She went on to explain the surgery is laparoscopic and exploratory for complete evaluation of the abdominal cavity. The endometriosis lesions are excised, or removed, from the surfaces of the organs, wherever they may be. The success rate was over 95 percent for complete excision and curative. Curative?! No one had dared to use that word with me yet! The office was so professional and organized, it wasn't long before I had all my medical records and copies of all my imaging sent to their chief surgeon for review.

By this time, woven somewhere in between all my gynecological visits and hospitalizations, a new diagnosis of ileitis had crept its way into my medical profile. Although my chronic pain had always claimed its stay on the right side of my lower abdomen, there had been something different about it. They determined I was going through bouts of ileitis — simply an inflammation of the ileum, the third portion of the small intestine, after the duodenum and jejunum, to be exact. It's the last stop right before the cecum, and it's where the large intestine begins. An intersection of sorts, located conveniently in our right lower abdomen, surrounded by several important neighbors, most notably our appendix. This little guy is theorized to be vestigial, the nicer way of saying a useless remnant of our evolutionary process. It was useful to our primitive ancestors and somewhere along the way lost its purpose, except it still sticks around in our genetic development as human beings. Regardless, I promise I'm going somewhere with this. As for my ileum, it felt like it was on fire every day.

Needless to say, I needed more answers. It took me mere seconds before I realized what that wave of emotion was, the one I felt during the phone conversation. It was hope. I held on to that hope with every strength that I had.

KINDNESS BREEDS KINDNESS

*I*n the middle of all this chaos — doctor's appointments, bone marrow biopsies and hospitalizations — I decided one day that I needed to do something with myself. It was an epiphany moment. My academics were on hold, and work and bed rest were not quite enough for me. I needed something meaningful to keep me occupied, motivated and distracted. "Aha!" I thought. "I'll plan a fundraiser!"

There was no turning back from that moment. Once I set my mind to it, I was planning a fundraiser for endometriosis awareness. What was supposed to be a small gathering of friends and family became a very large event with canopies, catering, live music, imprinted tote bags and many, many supportive friends and family.

I got in touch with the Endometriosis Research Center, also known as ERC, and expressed my interest in raising money toward its mission of raising awareness, advocacy, education, support and giving every victim a voice. I was so committed to the cause, it didn't matter. Something had to be done. This was my way of coping. I needed to help others. We could figure this out together.

I was connected with their executive director, Michelle Marvel. She was absolutely amazing. She guided me every step of the way. Next thing I knew, I was shopping around for a caterer willing to do a fundraiser gig at a low cost in exchange for business exposure! I was bargaining left and right. There were so many details I didn't consider when I first set out to complete this mission. At this stage of the game, it didn't matter. The process of organizing the fundraiser brought me back to earth, in a sense. It gave me a sense of purpose. The more I accomplished and checked off my list, the more determined I was to kick endo's ass.

The planning process kept me busy. Every time I thought I was close to the finish line, I had something else to unravel and piece together. But it was all coming together, and I found a perfect location: a local park that was centrally located on a main road and close to home. It was the perfect spot that offered everything we needed — picnic tables, a small area where food could be served and plenty of space for people to walk around and mingle. I called the parks and recreation department to reserve the space for our humble gathering. They had very few available dates, but one of them was Labor Day weekend. I took it and started advertising the event: Fly with the Endo Angels, September 3, 2006. My Uncle Steve is a musician and was gracious enough to supply us with great live entertainment. It was all coming together.

Promotion items included a tote bag with the name of the event, a photo of the Endo Angel used by the ERC and the name of our sponsors. Yes, I had sponsors! Family, close friends and local businesses contributed funds for planning. My loyal place of employment and second family, Arlington Dog & Cat Hospital, donated enough to earn a co-host title. My coworkers got together and pooled some money, securing a spot on the sponsors list. It's times like these that reveal who your true people are. I have been very fortunate to have a very large network of friends and support groups. I always have. It's because of this solid, continually growing network that I'm able to truly keep the sincere and devoted by my side. The insincere and the undevoted? We'll talk about those a little further down.

September third will always remain a special day for

me. I remember waking up that morning and hoping the weather forecasters would be wrong about a Nor'easter heading our way! I had no choice but to call around and order some canopies for some last-minute planning in case Mother Nature decided to grace us with a heavy rain shower. The skies looked pretty questionable, but that didn't get in the way. Rain or shine, this event was on. The yellow ribbon is the official endometriosis awareness color, so I decorated the picnic tables with yellow table covers, strategically placed sunflowers as the centerpieces and provided yellow ribbons for people to display proudly.

It was almost hard to believe the time had come. Now to greet the guests as they came in. Nothing would prepare me for how many people came through. My face was almost numb from smiling all day. There I was, surrounded by the most important people in my life, supporting me and a cause so near to my heart. We raised $11,000 for the Endometriosis Research Center that day. It was so amazing. It was almost amazing enough to allow me to forget what was coming up three days later in Atlanta, Georgia. I had scheduled my excision surgery and was flying down with my mother the next morning.

IT'S ALL RELATIVE

*T*repidation is a good word that comes to mind. I was facing surgery in a different state, where I would need to stay for several days to recover before I could travel again. There were so many unknowns. During the process of scheduling the surgery and speaking with the surgeon about my case, he had expressed his concern for my ileitis. With his experience, he suspected the reason behind the ileitis was invasion of endometrial lesions. If this were true, this would mean my endometriosis was spreading and working its way up my body. He explained the only way to know for certain was to examine the integrity of the ileum and other organs directly during the surgery. Before I could even finish my question in my head of what this would mean, he answered: I would be at risk of needing an intestinal resection. His words pierced through me. It was possible I would be leaving Atlanta not just without endo, but without a portion of my intestinal tract, and who knows what else. These words haunted me every day until surgery. All I could do was wait and pray.

The morning of the surgery, the doctor approached my mother and me with a very important decision I'd need to make prior to anesthesia. His question was what would be my decision if the endometriosis was severe enough to warrant a hysterectomy. There I was, a 22-year-old facing the decision of a possible hysterectomy and intestinal resection. My mother was faced with this plaguing question, as she would be the one the surgeon would be talking to during the surgery if there was a concern. I asked her to please tell him no hysterectomy. It was too permanent of a decision while I was so young. I got on the surgery gurney and was wheeled away. I had no way of knowing what to expect when I woke up from anesthesia. I looked at my mother as they took me away and saw the look of fear in her eyes with tears in mine.

The verdict: I was able to keep my uterus and ovaries, and even my ileum. The endometrial lesions had indeed invaded my intestinal tract, but the surgeon was able to salvage my intestine. He did make it clear that it was a very close call and the lesions had started to penetrate through. Wish I could say the same for my appendix. Endometrial lesions had taken it over enough to the point that it needed to be removed. Adios appendix. I don't miss you a bit. Thank you for taking the brunt of it. My ileum means so much more to me.

I was so happy about this news, it didn't even matter that I could barely sit up with soreness. I spent one night in the hospital and was cleared the next morning. My mother and I stayed at a local hotel for a few nights, so I could recover some more before traveling. The post-operative pain proved to be challenging. The carbon dioxide gas used to inflate my abdomen was still working its way around my abdomen, trying to find its way out. But you know what? It didn't matter. I had just had excisional surgery with an exceptional surgeon, my uterus and ovaries were still inside of me and my ileum was a happy camper. I was heading home soon and looking forward to feeling better in the next few weeks. What else could I ask for? It could have been worse. It's all relative, and I considered myself lucky.

ENDO WARRIOR COMING THROUGH

*M*y post-op recovery was smooth. I was actually pain free. As much as this delighted me, it was only short lived. About two months later, things started to change. I was having flashbacks — fear, anxiety and denial all crept back in. Was this pain just temporary or a figment of my imagination? It must be. I just had surgery! I said adios to endo and my appendix! Yet the pain was undeniable. I knew it well. I called the office with my concerns, but they advised me I would need to return to Atlanta. I felt myself starting to spiral. Why is this happening? I did everything right. I tried very hard to keep calm and not jump to conclusions. There are other possibilities, I'm sure, I told myself.

My gut told me to get on the internet and research. Even though I felt like I had exhausted all options, I continued to search and search and search, until it happened. I found a specialist in New York City. Wait, NYC? That's right here. Why didn't I find this before?

I still don't know the answer to that, but I didn't spend too much of my energy on it since I was gifted with yet another option. My only focus was to get into that office and get answers. Little did I know this visit would change my life forever.

It was right before Christmas, and I headed into New York City. My Aunt Lurdes met up with me at the doctor's office for support. I knew I had to prepare myself for every possible outcome. Endometriosis is not typically visible on an ultrasound; however, after the exam, the doctor knew exactly what was going on and what I needed. I was floored at his skills. I experienced a dichotomy between my fear and a sense of strange calmness I felt around Dr. Kanayama. I had just met him, yet I felt completely confident I was exactly where I needed to be.

I sat down in his office to discuss the examination results. He was very professional and clear. He reported: "Even though you just had surgery, your endometriosis has returned." My heart skipped a beat, but I kept quiet. His concern was apparent as he explained that this quick return of the disease indicated a rapid relapse, and that was not typical. This did not mean the previous surgery was not done correctly, since all it takes is a tiny speck of endo lesion left behind, and it can spread like wildfire. I knew my previous surgeon did a great job, and I was very grateful for his time, dedication and help. If it weren't for him, my intestines would still be at risk. However, that was in the past. Now, I needed to focus on what my next step would be. Turns out my next step was another surgery.

Three weeks later, on January 11, 2007, I was prepped and wheeled away on a gurney again. Déjà vu. Except this time, it would be my last surgery. I had a much rougher recovery this time around, but I kept the end goal in mind. I was positive this would be it. I felt I had landed in the right hands.

By this time, I had been out of school for about a year and a half. The next semester was set to start the week of January 20. Dr. Kanayama kept reminding me that I had just undergone a major abdominal surgery and needed at least eight weeks of recovery at home. I didn't doubt this at all, except I had reached my limit and decided to go back to class, whether I was recovered or not. Another classic example of my persistence. Once I set my mind to something, there's no stopping me. It had become clear that this battle with endo was most likely not going to be cut and dried, nor short lived. If this were the case, I might as well continue my education while I continued to fight.

Besides, it was positive mental stimulation and gave me alternative things to focus on, so I could keep my mind active. Or at least this is what I told myself to justify my decision. It worked.

My goal of going to veterinary school was still as fervent as before; in fact, focusing on my career goals supplied the additional fuel I needed to keep on moving forward. Hence, my inner endo warrior rose up and made its appearance, once again.

I bulldozed through. The first few weeks after surgery were torturous, to say the least. It took a good six weeks before I felt more comfortable getting around, yet I was attending class, still going to work, doing all the normal day-to-day things that made me feel like a person again. I'm not saying I recommend this at all. Please don't do anything that will jeopardize you.

The main reason I was able to endure the first month of post-operative recovery while still being active is simply because, by this time, my pain tolerance was so high. I know, not exactly something to strive for. But it was my reality. Gone were the days where I stayed in bed, wondering where my life was leading me. I chose to lead myself, and if this meant taking the brunt for a month after surgery so I could kick-start my education back up again, then so be it.

My eight-week recheck with Dr. Kanayama was a big turning point for me. I was still feeling pretty good. I wasn't feeling any unusual pain outside of what would be expected with surgery. I went in with positive vibes — and came out with positive vibes! The ultrasound revealed all my organs were much happier without those evil endo lesions, there was minimal scar tissue formation, and my ovaries and uterus were all happy as clams. All was right in the world.

If my story were like a novella that continued to turn down the same dreary path it had before, I would experience a dramatic turn of events right about now. But I didn't. My happy ovary clams stayed merry and reverted back to their normal function for several months before I felt different again. Except this time, the discomfort I felt was not like the endo pain I experienced before. Nonetheless, it was there. But I didn't panic. I kept myself calm and called the doctor's office for a recheck. I had gotten a taste of what it felt like to feel like a "normal" girl again. It was difficult for me to even fathom backpedaling to the endo days. So I kept myself distracted and didn't allow my mind to wander. If only it were that simple.

The moment of truth was here. I almost didn't

want to look at the ultrasound image, but I did. What I saw on my right ovary was a giant cyst. It was ginormous. I was surprised I didn't feel more pain with that thing in me! It was the size of a softball. I remember it measured close to eight centimeters. Flabbergasted, I looked at Dr. Kanayama, and I'm sure he realized I already knew what I was looking at by the expression on my face. I was mainly stunned at the size of it. I almost wanted to name it, like a small pet. Despite this finding, I still was not alarmed. In fact, it didn't really faze me. I started listing the positives: the pain (up until then) was tolerable for me, and there was still no endo. Again, it could have been worse. Remember, it's all relative.

The biggest risk of the cyst was, of course, that it could rupture at any time. Dr. Kanayama advised me that surgery wasn't necessary at that time, especially since I had just had one. He prescribed bed rest until the creature could reabsorb on its own through the following month, primarily to avoid rupture. His recommendation was not too surprising. But neither was my noncompliance.

By this point, I was so over bed rest, I continued on with my life as usual. I wish I could tell you that it didn't rupture. It ruptured, but I still conquered. The discomfort was then a much more consistent and sharper pain. I could almost feel the fluid swishing in my abdomen. This pain was enough to definitely stop me in my tracks. But I dealt with it. I would stop for a few seconds and brace myself. If I happened to be around anybody or talking to someone at work, I would nonchalantly bite the inside of my cheek and squeeze whatever it was I had in my pocket at the time and move on with my day.

At this time, I wasn't exactly sure what this meant long term. I figured I'd get through this one, enjoy the fact that I had still eluded endo and, once again, move on. It turned out — despite being on birth control pills to manage my hormone levels, keep endo away and hopefully suppress the growth of these giant ovarian cysts — every few months, another cyst would rear its ugly head. My cysts would form and grow on my right ovary. They would rupture, I'd deal, they'd heal, and I'd move on. This tango went on for quite some time, at least four or five years on a regular basis. It became part of my norm. It was far from being a great norm. If that was the worst of it, then so be it. This became my mantra. I dealt with it.

I continued on with my courses and graduated from Montclair State in 2009 with my degree in biology and English literature. This was a big deal. I finally made it. Four months later, I would be on my way to Ross University School of Veterinary Medicine in Saint Kitts, West Indies. This would mark a very clear end to a very difficult chapter in my life and the beginning of a brand new one … in the Caribbean.

A WHOLE NEW WORLD

*I*t was all new. All of it. There was an authentic excitement for leaving everything behind and starting all over again. The figurative feeling of leaving all those hurdles behind as I flew away to live in a different country for a few years just felt right. I had worked very hard to get to vet school, and I knew what I was up against. In a sense, after defeating endo, I felt invincible. The physical and emotional difficulty of overcoming endometriosis had, without a doubt, changed me forever. I can't help but wonder who I'd be today if I hadn't been obligated to navigate such challenging circumstances. Only when you truly look fear in the face do you realize your own strength. It humbles you.

If I wasn't humbled enough, Saint Kitts made sure I was. I took that leap of faith without even looking back. After what I had been through, taking risks was a whole different ball game. I looked at it as, if I failed, so what? As long as I had my health, I could pick right back up and move on to the next. This mentality not only stuck with me through vet school and into my first years of practice, but it's still with me. If it weren't for this attitude, I wouldn't be where I am today, and I'm sure this mindset will continue to guide me to whatever will be coming my way in future years. You never know what life will bring you, but whatever it is, accept it with open arms. The more we accept change, the more opportunities come our way. The more we don't focus on what other people are thinking, the more we can grow and be as diverse as possible. The more we put ourselves first, the more we learn to love ourselves, and the more others will respect you for who you are — the rest is magic.

Living in a foreign country for almost three years had its ups and downs, kind of like a roller coaster ride. Gee, this sounds familiar. The fluctuations of up and down, back and forth, didn't bother me a bit.

Caribbean islands don't have the luxuries of America. Electric outages occurred daily here, and we quickly learned how to improvise. It didn't take long for us to realize if we planned a visit to the supermarket on a Monday, the shelves would be practically cleared of any contents, especially the bread! This makes sense when we considered the weekly shipment of products arrived on Tuesdays, and until they got a new shipment, they couldn't restock any items. Most of the student body experienced island transportation. We purchased a recycled and recirculated vehicle that was over ten years old and could be lovingly characterized as a rusted piece of tin. Every single day, one of us would need a ride to campus because having our cars in the shop was inevitable. It would be negligent of me if I did not mention the carnivorous centipedes that would invade our apartments and posed a threat to our flesh, all the time.

Despite these entertaining occurrences, I adjusted pretty easily to the way of life in St. Kitts. I was so focused on the fact that I finally made it to vet student status, everything else just fell into place. What did anything else matter? I was very aware of my risk. There I was with minimal medical assistance nearby. The most common reaction from others when they hear I am a veterinarian (after the gasp) is, "I hear vet school is very hard. " Well, ain't that the truth. But focus and determination is the key. I knew vet school was not going to be a walk in the park, but neither was what I had just gone through with endo. If that's what life is going to be, one challenge after another, then I chose to embrace it and keep moving forward. By default, I kept setting the bar higher and higher.

It was in St. Kitts that I met and rescued my girl, Stella. For those of you who know me well, you know Stella has been my other half and loyal friend for many years. Stella was a mutt stray found deep in the rainforest of St. Kitts, roped to a tree with no food or water, starving away. She was taken in by Ross University, and this is where I came across her one day during one of our labs. She and I had an immediate connection. With my upcoming island departure a few months later, I offered to adopt her, and the rest is history. Yet another risk I didn't think twice about. Once I knew I could take her with me to the states, I didn't hesitate to sign the adoption papers. I knew I would figure it out, period. So for the last eight years, Stella has been with me through it all, and I intend to keep her happy for as long as I can. Jackson, her sidekick, is a Floridian humane society rescue that came into my life last year. Even though he didn't have to fly across a body of water to get here, he was also a spontaneous decision. Once I met him, I knew he was meant to be with us.

My point is: regardless of the risk I was taking, once again, the newly primed me didn't give it a second thought. I continued to have my share of ovarian cysts throughout my time spent churning away at vet school. But simply, I made it through, time after time. I was diligent and made sure I visited Dr. Kanayama in New York when I went home on my breaks. With each visit, I returned back to St. Kitts with a smile and feeling reassured. I had everything I needed. I was enrolled in a reputable veterinary school curriculum, in a place where I could feed my hunger for adventure and different cultural experiences, and, most of all, I was surrounded by a large group of supportive friends that I would gladly and lovingly refer to as my Island Family. I met these guys on day one of moving to the island, and they've been in my life since. I couldn't imagine my life without my experiences at Ross University.

My Island Family just celebrated the 10th anniversary of our move to St. Kitts. It's unbelievable to think a decade has gone by. Despite the number of years, that group is still in my life to this day. We may not see each other every day, but we know where we fit into each other's lives, and no matter how much time has gone by without seeing one another, our friendship remains. As we sprinkle the United States from the East to West Coast, somehow we always manage to find time for meetups, weddings, weekend trips and conferences.

That's true friendship. Something that is so difficult to come by in a world where reputation, jealousy, insecurities, toxic people and competition tend to take precedence, especially in our current age of social media. If you really care deeply about someone, your support should be unwavering, not inconsistent or only when convenient for you. In an age where life fulfillment is defined by external factors, such as what others think of you and expect of you, true happiness comes from within. I know this isn't the first time you've heard this message, and it won't be the last. So do yourself a favor and genuinely think about it. Your inner beast signifies change, freedom and growth, and it's yearning to be let out. Now take a deep breath and release it.

Part Two:
Balance and Harmony

REPEAT AFTER ME

*Y*ou all have a warrior within you. If you're reading this and you don't specifically have endometriosis, you still have a warrior within you. This isn't just about women who are currently experiencing the challenges of endometriosis; it's about any human being's ability to rise up when facing life challenges. You can be a man or a woman, young, middle-aged or elderly — it doesn't matter. You can be facing endo, IBD, diabetes, heart disease, Crohn's disease, kidney failure, depression, cancer … the big-picture message here is that if you don't stand up for yourself and believe you *will* overcome, no one else will do it for you. It needs to come from you. Having a support system — family and friends — is so important when trekking through the muddy waters, but no one can really get you out of that thick mud but yourself. You need to find courage within yourself. Reach deep down and uncover that warrior because it's just waiting there to be discovered.

We know not everything has a definitive cure. How many times did I have to read or hear there's no cure for endometriosis? Yet here I am, in the flesh, endo free for almost 13 years now. When I stop to think of this, it's still very surreal to me.

What's my secret? Everything in this book is my secret. There is no one answer. It's a grand combination of medical, mind, body and spirit. The medical has all to do with advocating for yourself and your own body. Listen to what your heart is telling you when you're presented with treatment options and facing decisions. Make sure you feel like you have a connection with your doctor and that you feel like you're being heard. Do your research; make educated decisions.

Beyond the medical, taking care of your mind, body and spirit is a real thing. This isn't just something you see printed on T-shirts and the front windows of yoga studios. There's something very real and tangible about truly taking care of yourself in ways beyond just taking your daily vitamins and taking appropriate prescriptions.

A healthy being requires balance and harmony. I can't help but flash back to my first veterinary school course in physiology, which laid the foundation for my future practice. To this day, I can remember my professor explaining homeostasis — simply the state of maintaining stability within an organism. As doctors, our main task is to keep our patients stable and functional. That's it. All those years of medicine, classes and practically drowning in study material boil down to our ability to keep patients stable. When someone is hit by a car or some other traumatic event that results in hemorrhage or severe blood loss, unless we can control that bleeding, it doesn't matter if the patient is still able to breathe or not. They can breathe all they want, but there's no blood transferring oxygen to the body. In order to reestablish homeostasis, the bleeding needs to be controlled while maintaining a patent airway.

We all take for granted the thousands of intricate processes that occur within our bodies, every second of our lives. It's not very often we sit there and think about exactly what our pancreas is doing with insulin to continually keep our blood sugar stable or how our blood pressure is continually being regulated with intrinsic baroreceptors. How about how our temperature primarily sticks around 98.6 degrees Fahrenheit or how our immune system never stops the surveillance necessary to keep us alive day to day. Ever wonder how our breathing almost seems involuntary?

That's our body's way of keeping homeostasis as it balances oxygen and carbon dioxide. You don't even have to think about it! Fascinating stuff. Without homeostasis, the body is imbalanced. Imbalance equals disease.

Our bodies are gifts. You only get one, so treat it nicely. So many of us take our bodies for granted. Every living being on this earth shares the demons of insecurity, fear and deep internal issues to a certain extent. Once again, we're all human. This is where going to therapy, focusing on our sense of self, taking classes, practicing mindfulness — you know, life balance stuff — will not let you down. I've learned seeking these options and integrating them into my daily existence is a significant part of keeping myself balanced and harmonized. It means you're prioritizing you —you're putting yourself first.

For example, I commit myself to the same yoga class every Sunday morning. I show up at the same time, same place, with the same group of lady yogis. It's my way of liberating myself from just about everything. It's the time I can disconnect from the world as I enjoy my weekly quiet time on my mat. It's the one time my phone is turned off and set aside. It is time for me. Whatever stresses I bring to the mat with me that week transform into lesser priorities, as this environment allows me to focus on putting things into perspective. Okay — it may have been a stressful week, but when I'm there, I'm surrounded by a great group of women. I feel safe, I have my health and I hold the power to mold my day into whatever I'd like it to be. What else can you ask for? Everything else just simply becomes background noise.

However, we can't always just disconnect. We also have to connect with the world at times, and we have to face our fears and anxieties head-on. When you do this, try to put your pride aside and forget about shame. Embrace your vulnerability. It may feel like a losing battle, but really your courage is step one to victory. No one else will get you there but you. While you are facing your fears and anxieties, repeat the mantra below.

Repeat after me:
Balance and harmony are my friends
:::Breathe:::
I need balance and harmony
:::Breathe:::
I have an inner warrior
:::Breathe:::
Put myself first

:::Breathe:::

I am grateful for …

Now that we've unpacked the importance of balance and harmony within a healthy being, let's go over some ways I have found very useful in achieving this blissful state.

NUTRITION DOES A BODY GOOD

The world of medicine and pharmacy is a very important one. It's what our standard healthcare system is based on. While medicine plays such an integral role in disease management and pain relief, I believe it is just as necessary to open our minds and incorporate the world of the "other" things out there, like nutrition, awareness of the mind-body connection, physical exercise, yoga, rehabilitation, energy healing, maintaining qi flow with acupuncture, tai chi, mindfulness and meditation, breathing exercises, herbal treatment, massage ... the list can go on and on.

As a result of what I went through with hormone therapy and because I had reached my limit with doctors throwing prescriptions for pain medications at me, I found myself gravitating toward the alternative realm. I use the word alternative here loosely, meaning anything other than standard pharmaceutical medications/therapy. These alternative therapies became such a core part of my life, I even began integrating them into my own practice of veterinary medicine. My patients, whatever ailment they present for, are all gifted with the options of alternative medicine. My treatment plans often include anything from medicine/drugs, supplements, targeted nutrition, acupuncture, physical rehabilitation/therapeutic modalities, chiropractic and herbs. And it all works beautifully.

While I was actively battling endo, I had a hunger for more information (no pun intended). So I got back on the internet and bought a stack of books. I focused on nutrition first — so many conditions can be managed by what we eat. We hear it all the time: we are what we eat. Yet nutrition is rarely discussed as a significant option and recommendation when it comes to medical management of almost anything. Maybe it's mentioned in passing when it comes to things like high blood pressure or diabetes, but how often is it truly explained and prioritized within a treatment plan? It's so crucial to feed our bodies appropriate nutrients for mental clarity, maintaining a healthy weight, fueling energy and, most importantly, avoiding inflammation. Inflammation equals pain.

Endometriosis pain is a direct consequence of inflammation. We know there are certain foods and drinks that contribute to inflammation, known as pro-inflammatory. Inflammation is a complex molecular cascade of events that involves the release of cytokines. Put simply, cytokines are messenger signaling cells that are released by the immune system. In functionality, the process of inflammation is an integral part of our immune system or host defense. It's one of the immune system's weapons used to combat injury and trauma, protect cells and ultimately promote healing. Just as with anything in life, it is very possible to have too little or too much inflammation.

My own personal strategy was to tackle the things that I had direct control over right now to help kick endo's butt. Knowing I have every control over what I place in my mouth and into my body, every single day, I turned to nutrition. Did I expect nutrition to single-handedly defeat endo for me and all my troubles would be over? No. But I did expect eating well to help manage my pain level and nourish my body with the necessary nutrients to keep moving forward, physically and mentally. Let's just consider a brief list of things we eat that are known to be pro-inflammatory.

- **Sugar, sugar, sugar.** Our favorite sweet friend.

Sugar and high fructose corn syrup are the two most common **added** sugars we see in our diets. This means they're present in things like desserts, ice cream, doughnuts, pastries, puddings, cakes, soda, energy drinks, sports drinks, candy and condiments and sauces, like ketchup, barbecue sauce, hoisin sauce, teriyaki sauce, salad dressings and relish. Even yogurt and granola. The list can go on and on. Don't forget the sugar added to your coffee.

- **Artificial trans fats.** There's no way around this one aside from just stating the obvious. Fried and fast foods are your culprits here.

- **Refined carbohydrates.** Pasta, white bread, pizza dough, pastries, white flour, desserts ... Ouch, it hurts to keep going.

- **Processed meat/processed foods.** Snacks, chips, crackers, deli meat, hot dogs.

Depressing, isn't it? Everyone's favorite foods down the drain. Please don't feel like you need to isolate yourself and live on seeds and nuts for the rest of your life. The big picture here is to be mindful of what you put into your body. There are so many resources and books on nutrition, diets and recipes. It's very possible to indulge in delicious meals while still doing your body good. (Believe me, I am a mega-foodie.) Write out a doable, gradual plan for yourself. Don't put pressure on yourself, and be realistic with your goals. Any positive step toward being mindful of your body and health is something to celebrate. It's a big deal! You've already started — you're reading this book.

Naturally, while there are foods that are pro-inflammatory, there are conversely healing foods and nutrients with anti-inflammatory properties. These are the guys we want to focus on. A planned anti-inflammatory diet is geared toward minimizing the inflammatory cascade, blocking those unnecessary cytokines and accomplice molecules while supplying your body with the nutrients it needs. Let's dive in.

- **Berries.** Pick one! Strawberries, blueberries, blackberries ... they're all delicious, rich in antioxidant properties and conquer inflammation.

- **Broccoli.** Yum. I know it gets a bad reputation, but it's not the worst tasting vegetable out there, and it offers so much nutrition that keeps those bad cytokines at bay.

- **Avocados.** Who wouldn't want vitamins C, E, K and B6, niacin, folate, potassium, magnesium and omega-3 fatty acids all in one delicious package?

- **Leafy greens**. Spinach, kale, collards … you name it, these greens make tasty salad beds or are great on their own, too.

- **Omega-3 fatty acids.** I'm a huge fan of omega-3s and recommend them continuously to my own four-legged patients. Naturally anti-inflammatory, they benefit skin, joints, eyes, kidneys and the uterus. They're found in foods like salmon, tuna and mackerel. If you're not a fish person, there are thousands of supplements readily available. Walnuts, chia seeds and kidney beans can also be part of the omega-3 team.

- **Green tea.** This was my personal favorite. Once I dove into the world of tea, there was no turning back. The healing properties and benefits of green tea alone are mind-blowing. With its bioactive compounds and powerful antioxidant properties, green tea is proven to reduce free radicals (the product of cell damage), thereby creating an environment of happy, healthy cells. Green tea has been shown to

  o reduce your risk of common diseases, including heart disease, diabetes, high cholesterol, stroke and even the big C word —

cancer

- o   aid in metabolism, fat burning and weight loss
- o   reduce inflammation anywhere in the body
- o   benefit digestive health and mental health
- o   fight skin cancer by helping to protect against UV rays and repair damaged DNA;
- o   reduce age-related changes.

Isn't it magical? All it takes is some boiled water and a tea bag. I will admit, it was an acquired taste for me. I drank it straight up without adding any sugar or sweeteners. But I was so determined to reap the benefits of such an easily accessible and affordable option, I learned to love it. I drank four or five cups of tea per day at my worst. To this day, I'm known to have my tea in the morning or any chance I get. Why not?

Speaking of drinking, don't underestimate the power of hydration. Water is your friend, and it's a basic element that is absolutely necessary for proper bodily function. Carry a refillable water bottle with you. It will make a world of a difference, and your body will thank you with improved skin on top of other health benefits.

NO EXTRA BAGGAGE PLEASE — BEING MINDFUL

*S*urvival is a tricky thing. In our ancestral Neanderthal days, not only did our predecessors rely on the fight-or-flight response to survive, they relied on each other. The fight-or-flight response is a physiologic chemical response within our bodies that gives us the juice needed to run from that tiger or enemy with a spear. Granted, regardless of the evolutionary transformation in our ancestral DNA, when it comes to things like our appearance, our size and our stance, these changes failed to translate into the design of our sympathetic nervous system.

You know that feeling you get when you're stressed all of a sudden, like you're feeling threatened in some way? That is our fight-or-flight response. This response is intended to help us through legit life-threatening events; however, due to our busy, chaotic, high-pressure modern lifestyles we live today, everything is a threat to us all the time. We are continuously in survival mode. Nothing is ever enough. This is called stress. And it's no bueno. No bueno at all.

Wouldn't it be absolutely amazing if there was a simple switch we could use to turn off stress? Wouldn't that be more practical? We would certainly all be walking around much healthier, no doubt. Chronic stress leads to the disease worsening. It's that simple. It's a massive epidemic within our working society, yet it's not important enough for people to stop and reflect on what they're doing to themselves. Why would we? It's exactly what society expects of us, right?

Yet, we need to learn to manage our stress.

We can talk about how important it is to nourish your body with proper nutrition and keep yourself active with exercise, but the meat and potatoes of balance and harmony is your mental health. We absolutely want our muscles to feel strong and healthy, our cardiovascular system to be as efficient as it can be and for our organs to keep plugging away. They make up our physical existence. However, let's not forget who reigns over the domain and is responsible for our physical wellness and stability — none other than your mind. The big kahuna of it all. The mind-body connection is no joke. It's powerful, it's scientific and it's one of the single most important contributing factors to our well-being. Dr. John Sarno was a brilliant physician and professor who became known for his studies and pioneering the revelation of the mind-body connection. He has written several books that I believe are well worth your time and investment.

Simply put, our minds dominate our physical state. The term used is psychosomatic. Psyche means mind. Somatic means body. Thoughts, emotions, beliefs and attitudes set the stage. It's a complex, closely-knit interrelationship between three major body systems — the nervous system, endocrine system and immune system. Our whole existence relies on the intimate relationship between this trio. Think about it. When you feel nervous, where do you feel it the most? We say we have butterflies in our stomach. When you feel highly stressed or like you're in immediate danger, you feel your heart pounding within your chest, increasing the amount of blood and subsequently oxygen into your body, so you're ready to face your incoming threat. Remember the fight-or-flight response we spoke of earlier? It makes sense when you think about it, right?

There are a plethora of neural pathways by which our brain connects to our organs and the musculoskeletal system. Think of them as highways that serve as conduits, allowing transportation back and forth. This communication between the central nervous system and the peripheral nervous system is crucial for our survival and function and is accomplished primarily through the intricate work of neurotransmitters. I like to think of these guys as the life juice of our bodies. Our hearts rely on messages that guide heart rate and contraction, our adrenal glands need to know how much cortisol to pump out, our muscles rely on messages that tell them to contract and move, and even our pupils receive signals that lead to dilation or constriction! And these are only a few basic examples.

Most of you have likely come across the words *serotonin*, *dopamine*, *acetylcholine* and *norepinephrine*. That's because, although there are hundreds of them, these are the big neurotransmitters. If you're going to look into some of these, serotonin is a good one. It plays a large role in the body, regulating mood, digestion, sleep, memory and sexual desire. It can be referred to as the "happy chemical." In the brain, it has a hand in our mood, anxiety level and, you guessed it, happiness. Depression has been linked to low levels of serotonin, but it still remains unclear whether low serotonin causes depression or the other way around. Despite the fuzzy lines of interpretation, we know a lot of antidepressants are targeted at elevating serotonin levels in our brain. So there must be something to it. Now let's take it a step further. If low levels of serotonin can be blamed for so many unpleasant moods and ill effects, then what do they say helps elevate serotonin in the brain?

- nutrition, diet, supplements
- getting enough sleep
- managing stress levels
- getting puppy kisses (had to squeeze that one in there)

Starting to sound familiar? What it boils down to is taking care of yourself, a.k.a. maintaining balance and harmony. I know it's much easier said than done, but please trust me when I say it can very possibly be done.

So we've covered nutrition and eating healthy. Getting enough sleep is also a given. We as human beings sleep for a reason. Sleep is meant to be a restorative period for our bodies and minds. Ironically, serotonin levels have a direct influence on our sleeping patterns, as does dopamine. Although there are several factors that can affect one's sleep quality, I personally believe we all need to shut our brains off. Period.

The sleep cycle has different stages: 1,2,3 and REM. These stages are characterized by different patterns of brain wave activity by measuring frequency and amplitude. In the early phases of Stage 1, alpha waves are produced. This means the brain is relaxed, yet awake. This is also when the subconscious mind awakens and unleashes every buried negative thought you could possibly have. It all comes barreling up to the surface. We reenact, reinvent, play and replay difficult events from our day. Sometimes we also imagine events that are going to take place. Tiring, isn't it? Enter mindfulness. This is where practicing mindfulness and controlling our thoughts can really go far. The subconscious mind is more powerful than it's given credit for. Because it is subconscious, we don't stop to think of its impact on our mental health. Meanwhile, it's continuously running in the background, incognito, with all its almighty power. These negative thoughts that reflect what you are afraid of have the highest potential to derail you. As you run through scenarios that haven't even occurred, you are putting those bad thoughts out there, and now they may very well happen. The negativity energy transmitted from your thoughts is a reality. The actual fearful unrealistic thoughts you are reeling through are the fantasy. Let that sit for a minute. In short, while you may think you are resting, as long as your subconscious is awake, you're not. Silencing the mind is a true art, and it takes practice, but it certainly isn't impossible. You just need to put your mind to it.

Although often implied with emotions and moods, stress in itself is the leading cause of practically everything: chronic inflammation, pain, any disease, cancer, you name it. Stress is a chemical reaction. Picture your ancestors again, fleeing from the saber-tooth tiger. Once again, the fight-or-flight response is meant to be a beneficial cascade of chemical triggers within the body that heighten our chances of survival when faced with danger. The adrenal glands receive the danger signals from the brain, and within seconds, cortisol and norepinephrine are churned out into the body. Your pupils dilate; your heart rate, breathing rate and blood pressure go up; and more glucose is dumped into your bloodstream for sustained energy. While cortisol and norepinephrine do a good job of kicking it up a notch, they also do just as splendid of a job of turning things down. Naturally, during a crisis, our digestive system, reproductive system and immune system, to name a few, are unnecessary (you certainly don't need them when running from a tiger). In short, stress suppresses our immune systems. When we're consistently in stress mode in response to our daily perceived "stresses," we put ourselves at mega-risk for diseases and conditions with no defense. Just think, do you think it's a coincidence you usually get sick when you're mostly run down, stressed and tired? Our immune systems literally keep us alive, every single day. Most pathogens we encounter every waking hour of our lives go unnoticed because our immune system neutralizes the threats incognito, and we move on with our lives. The loyal surveillance of our immunity humbly persists with its duties as much as it's allowed to — until cortisol comes barging in and shuts down the party. It's like the guest that just doesn't leave.

So, again, why is it that we torture ourselves time after time and remain prisoners to our own negative thought processes and stressful responses? Because the evil bandits need to be stopped and dealt with. We are humans. You need to stop and really reflect. What is it that really makes your heart happy? Only you can answer that. This is where we, as our own selves, need to step in and take control. Where do you begin? Love yourself first.

Managing stress comes right back to putting yourself first. What is it that keeps your stress level under control? Is it making time for that yoga class on a Wednesday night, taking a hot bath on a schedule to take the tension off and calm your mind, or maybe aromatherapy is what does the trick for you? Maybe it's all of the above. It could be something as simple as sitting in a dark room, in silence. Or watching a series you're so into, it allows you to forget the challenges from your day. On the other hand, it could be spending time with your kids and family with everything but silence. Whatever it is, allow yourself to do it. Own it and make it yours.

Part Three:
Love Yourself First

KNOW YOUR WORTH

" *L*ove yourself first, then everything else falls into line." This is a quote by the one-and-only, amazing Lucille Ball. There's so much truth to these words. You hear people saying this all the time, but what does it really mean? I'll admit, I personally have had a difficult time with the ambiguity of these three words. I mean, what do I really need to do to actually love myself? Are you saying I don't love myself? I thought I loved myself, but I guess not?

The answer is, there is no exact answer. This is one of those wishy-washy sentiments that is different for everyone. Personally, although it seemed complicated to me at first, and it took me a while to come to a conclusion on my own, loving myself means putting myself first. This has only been a realization for me in this past year. There's no growth without challenges, risks and failures. The more we get knocked down, the more swiftly we get back up the next time.

I definitely transformed during those few years when I was actively fighting endometriosis, repetitive ovarian cysts and fibromyalgia. I went from being an innocent 20-year-old focused on work and school to an adult facing tough medical decisions, advocating for myself, researching my own answers, planning a fundraiser for awareness, deciding to go back to school a couple of weeks after surgery and completely committing to my career as a veterinarian, all in quick succession. When that fire to survive and beat endometriosis lit up inside me, I knew I wasn't the same girl I had been just a few years before. Nothing would stand in my way. That same fire still lives inside me. It's like the Olympic torch. Even almost 15 years later, I find myself standing up for what I feel is appropriate and what I stand for. Some people may call it stubbornness; I call it dignity. When I reflect on how harrowing those days were and wonder who I would be if I didn't face those challenges, one thing is for sure: it prepared me for what was up next, in the next 15 years!

Still today, what I face each and every day prepares me for what's coming tomorrow and the rest of my life. The scariest part of looking back is seeing that once I felt home-free from endometriosis, it didn't end there. I still faced ovarian cysts and fibromyalgia. But these were more bearable for me because of my first experience with endo. And while they became a part of my life for some time, I conquered them, too. What didn't end were the challenges. Just when you think you're in the clear, another wake-up call is just around the corner.

Next came veterinary school and all the good and bad that came with it. After that? I was a practicing veterinarian facing the challenges vets face every day. And then? Still facing that challenge, I pursued my passion for improving the human-animal bond, while improving the quality of life of my furry patients. The challenges? Compassion fatigue, ethical debates, the pressures and responsibilities that come with being the veterinarian whose license is continually at risk, clients who take their own personal issues out on you and difficult and toxic coworkers who think gossip and drama are more interesting than focusing on patients or improving themselves. These challenges are so real within the veterinary world that we've seen a spike in the suicide rate among veterinarians. Every few months, we hear of yet another veterinarian suicide due to the immense stress and pressure that come with our responsibilities. It breaks my heart every time. This needs to change.

These are real-life issues that exist in almost every person's work-life or career, am I right? We spend over 90 percent of our time at work and immersed in our careers while everything else comes second, third and fourth. I understand our jobs and careers are necessary to be able to live our lives and support ourselves while giving us a sense of purpose, but when work is so stressful and toxic to our mental stability, what do we do then? What is the breaking point?

It is important to realize that no matter how much we would love to control our lives and fully take the steering wheel, life will always throw us curveballs. But, you can sure as hell control how you respond to the curveballs by preparing yourself mentally and nurturing your soul. This is why it's so crucial to love yourself first. Loving yourself means putting yourself first. When you put yourself first, you prioritize everything we have spoken about: eating healthily, exercising, practicing mindfulness, meditating, getting enough sleep, yoga, acupuncture, reiki, tai chi, massage therapy, practicing the art of saying no, setting boundaries and the like. It becomes your mission to be as balanced as you can be, whatever that looks like for you. I'm sure some of you are thinking this sounds too selfish. Well, go ahead and be selfish, then, if that's what it takes for you to take care of yourself. I don't think it's being selfish. In fact, I think it's being **selfless**.

The way I look at it, the more you put yourself first, the more you can help others or improve your life with others. Whether this means a happier, healthier and more balanced you to share with your significant other, your children, your family, your friends, your coworkers, your pets. Anyone that is determined enough to go the extra mile necessary to continually focus on their own health and well-being is not just doing it for their own sake, they're doing it for the sake of others. By loving yourself, you're able to love others even more.

Find your passion. What is it in life that completely allows you to be on cloud nine? It can be an adventure or something you do within the privacy of your own home — anything that fulfills your soul. Mine is travel, hands down. I cannot describe the feeling of going somewhere new; meeting new people; not knowing what the next day holds; and the anticipation of beauty, culture and appreciation of what this world has to offer. For me, exploring this world keeps me grounded. It brings me to life, every time. For you, it may be travel as well, or it may be something simple, such as canvas painting or listening to music with no one else around.

Regardless of what it is, these passions and escapes are so significant to our existence and goal of striving for balance and harmony. It's what we all need in order to offer the <u>best</u> version of ourselves.

What it means to love yourself:

- Setting boundaries
- Knowing your limits
- Saying no proudly (but nicely)
- Advocating for yourself
- Trusting in yourself and your abilities
- Eliminating toxic people around you, pronto!
- Truly knowing you *are* enough
- Putting an end to apologizing
- Finding your escape or happy place

Through trials and tribulations, with action comes confidence and courage, with confidence and courage come believing in yourself, and with believing in yourself comes self-love. You can either keep listening to what others think you should do, or you can take action and take the reins and do what makes *you* happy. Your choice.

SET YOUR BOUNDARIES AND DON'T BUDGE

*F*ocusing on mental health was tougher than focusing on nutrition! The main reason is that nutrition and lifestyle changes are something you adjust solely with yourself. Sure, maybe these changes can affect your significant other or may have some influence on how you do things with your children or family, but for the most part, it's a decision that is reliant solely on your own actions. In other words, you're not typically requesting anything of others, aside from support and understanding.

But with our mental health, we do have to include others and set boundaries. I feel so strongly about the subject of relationships and how we as individuals are affected by the people around us; it is important to really consider these upcoming thoughts and reflections. I have mentioned before, my personal evolution in these last 15 years has been steadily unabating. While the first decade after my successful surgery with Dr. Kanayama was spent keeping myself physically balanced and focusing my attention on pulling through vet school, the last five years or so have proven to be a different ballgame. It was only after graduation, and in practice, that I began to realize it's not quite enough to just eat, sleep and exercise well.

When working on maintaining life balance, many forget to analyze their social circle. Our interactions with the people around us contribute so much to the integrity of our thought processes. Ever feel an overwhelming feeling of heaviness or dullness when a negative person is present with you in the room? There are people who are known to be energy vampires. These energy suckers are draining and, not to mention, a negative influence on your self-preservation of balance. It is much more difficult to fight the pessimism that flows out of a toxic person than to resist it. Most don't know how to. Most don't even know it's happening!

Toxic people often can seem like an ordinary person. They can be found in the workplace (most commonly), within your circle of friends, in your neighborhood, at the grocery store, at the gym, essentially anywhere. These negative nellies can be known as drama queens/kings, gossipers, complainers, the perpetual victim, pessimists, those that are always on the defense — people who would much rather project their toxicity onto others versus looking inside them for growth and improvement. It's much easier to put someone else down than it is to work on our own insecurities, am I right? It's called blowing out someone else's candles. If you really stop to analyze social interactions or behavior around you for a few days, you may discover you have allowed toxic people into your life. Consider how many of these you can pick out. Typically, this works best in an environment you are in continuously, like work or school, versus with strangers on the street. There needs to be dialogue and interaction to be able to decipher these beings. But once you have recognized it, it'll be ubiquitous. Just try it.

Taking the time to recognize this is important because what it boils down to is our mental health is very dependent on our relationships with others. Yes, many of our thoughts and emotions are self-created, and we are very capable of self-sabotage. Some of us do it to ourselves on a daily basis; however, our interactions with others are also significant and should not be underestimated. In fact, our relationships with others are the foundation of most of our thought patterns, whether they're positive or negative. Taking a good look around us may just be one of the best things we can do for ourselves. If you stop to really think about this right now, I'm willing to bet there are at least a few people you could live without. Just take a minute.

Am I right? The funny part is, it's not even about the people you can live without. It's the people you *should* live without. It's so common and easy to overlook certain people's hurtful or negative behaviors because they're our friends. No one wants to cause tension with their friends. I get it. But my next question is, are they truly your friend? Answer this as truthfully as you can. Are they really your friend if they hurt your feelings time after time, show signs of jealousy and downplay your achievements, or are so pessimistic all the time it affects your own capability of moving on to positive things?

Don't underestimate the power of equity

We all know what it feels like to be the one that puts in more effort and energy into someone else, only to not receive the same in return.

Maybe you drop everything anytime someone needs a favor. Maybe you're thoughtful and buy them gifts because it makes you feel good. Maybe you listen to their constant complaining. Maybe you're a person they need to know to advance themselves in their own careers. But do they do the same for you? This is called equity. For any healthy relationship between two human beings to be possible, whether this is between friends, coworkers, significant others or family members, there needs to be equity. We want to know that we're reaping the same benefits as the amount of energy we're putting into someone else. At first, it may seem natural that one person does more than the other, and it's no big deal. With time, trust me, this imbalance rears will exhibit itself as resentment, frustration, hurt and, most of all, betrayal.

I have a lot to say when it comes to relationships and how they impact our lives. It can be another book on its own. We want to give everyone the benefit of the doubt. Sometimes it's so clear to others around us what is going on, but we don't see it ourselves. Yes, this falls into the territory of denial, but for me, even more so, it's that we want to believe and have hope that people will change. We put our capes on and are ready to be their superhero. We care so much about them, we want to help in any way we can. Eventually, we find out we're going around in circles. Any time there seems to be a prospect of improvement, a thoughtful gift appears, or a favor is completed with absolutely no reluctance, this must mean there are changes coming and we are on the right track! Or your not-so-loyal friend is purposely attempting to reel you back in, and the cycle starts all over again.

This may or may not sound familiar to many of you. If it's not, consider yourself lucky. The more in tune we are to these acts of manipulations, the clearer they become, and the better you can dodge them. This can be achieved by setting boundaries. I cannot stress how important this is. Set your expectations. It's up to you to decide how much of yourself you'd like to give to each individual person. Think of yourself as a pie with only so many slices available. Ask yourself, does this person deserve a piece of my pie? Is there something about them that you can't put your finger on, and your gut is setting off sirens? Listen closely and set your boundaries. These skills can be refined with practice. It just takes awareness.

Put yourself first. Once your boundary lines are clearly demarcated, those who are prone to take advantage will no longer have a leg to stand on. Their benefit is, poof, gone. Sure, you can help with a favor, but it won't be for a few days until you are able to. Take it or leave it. You'll be amazed at the changes you'll see.

My intention is certainly not to dictate how anyone conducts their friendships or any other relationships. Although, what I do know is not everyone taps into this reality very readily. Sometimes it can take years of circle after circle after circle to realize there is something the matter, and you are being walked all over, time and time again. My best advice is to pay attention. So often we're so focused on the obvious, we're missing the big picture. The warrior within you will appreciate the strides you've taken to eat healthily, exercise, meditate and do reiki and tai chi. But there will always be a piece missing from your warrior toolbox if you allow yourself to be taken advantage of, over and over again. Stick up for yourself, and everything else will fall into place.

Detox your circle. You will be so thankful you did.

Once you set boundaries, there's no turning back. This is because you start to realize how healthy it is to put your foot down and say, take me as I am. Accept who you are, flaws and all. No one is perfect. Who cares about being perfect? Who gets to decide what defines perfect, anyway? You want to be the best version of yourself you can be. When you embrace and accept this, everything else falls into place. Your outlook on life changes for the better. The energy you emanate now attracts positive people and situations. No more lingering around Debbie Downers who have their feet stuck in the mud. Move forward, and do what it is that makes *you* happy. Do me a favor. Please do not compare yourself to others. Just don't do it. Others are living their lives as they see fit. You live yours. What makes your heart beat a different beat?

Let's look at the definition of jealousy: stay away. That's my definition. Jealousy is a very potent thought or emotion felt when you feel a sense of inadequacy, fear, anger or helplessness. There is absolutely no use for jealousy in anyone's life. This would indicate a desire to possess something someone else has, whether it's a materialistic object, a characteristic or a life situation. I cannot think of one healthy reason why you would begin to even consider such rubbish. Instead of expending our precious energy on continuously analyzing the lives of others, that sacred energy can be applied to our own growth. Take your time and valuable thought processes and redirect them internally. Transform the negative emotion associated with jealousy that serves no positive purpose into the zest needed to accomplish those desires you're jealous of. Make things happen in your own life. Forget everyone else's lives. Don't be helpless, be **selfless**!

If someone is jealous of you, consider it a

compliment! I know we tend to get all worked up and defensive when we feel someone is invading our space with jealous intentions, but it only means they're not able to do what you do. They're incapable of coming up to your level, and once again, instead of working on themselves, they take you down with them. Detox.

Repeat after me: I am myself. I am enough. I value myself. My value is enough. The truth is, the more you learn to value yourself, the less you want to be around people who don't. It almost becomes addictive, in a good way. Once you know how liberating it feels to stick to your guns, no matter what comes your way, it's difficult not to. This is the sweet spot. It's the place to be. It just takes practice. In fact, you'll learn to spot a toxic person a mile away, and once they've shown you this quality, you won't even be willing to give them even a day to prove otherwise. Because you *will* know and you *will not* tolerate it. You honor your space and time too much to even give them a second thought. It's just not worth it.

Even though my journey that I outline here spans about 15 years, I've only figured this last part out in the last couple of years. Up until then, I had done my best with all the other goodies I've outlined. But this detoxing has been the most recent facet that I've been working on. In fact, I still am working on it as I write this. In my opinion, this is the most pivotal part. So if you're going to take any portion of this book to heart, I recommend you pay close attention to this one.

Before I move forward with this subject, it's important to point out that egotism equals insecurity. Anyone that blows out everyone else's candle so theirs can shine brighter is someone with deep-rooted insecurities, and they need help. Rather than looking inside themselves and working on their own flaws, it's much easier to knock everyone else down first. Everyone has experienced something similar to this in one way or another. I have personally faced a handful of people like this in the last five years. Time after time, each struggle wore me down.

As much as you feel compelled to help them, whether they're your friends, your family or your coworkers, you cannot do anything to change them. Trust me, I've been through this rodeo one too many times. They need to want to change and do the work themselves. As much as it hurts to turn away someone like this, it's the only way you can save yourself and set yourself free from their toxic grip. If it's a close friend or family member that you love, it can absolutely be heart-wrenching to feel like you're turning your back on them. But realize, if you don't leave them be, they are the ones turning their back on you, time after time after time. If your toxic person is a colleague at work, the best you can do is to be yourself and show your strengths and true potential. Take your self-worth and let it shine. I promise you, they'll eventually lose interest and move on to someone else. Once you put yourself first, you realize how easy it is to wall off the unwanted. This was precisely how I knew I had broken ground myself, just this past year. So you see, growth and self-love are perpetual processes with unexpected turns. At least it keeps things interesting.

MAKE IT CONTAGIOUS

*B*y this time, you've either connected with the things I've dubbed "life essentials" or not, or maybe somewhere in between. I really hope you have, at least enough to possibly trigger some different thought patterns that you have never considered before. Don't be afraid of being **selfless**. If you're not your own priority, how do you expect yourself to fully show up? How are you able to tackle life's challenges when you're incomplete yourself?

Start thinking of yourself as yet another human being with life struggles. There's nothing to be ashamed of. Kick shame to the curb. You will find that the positive thoughts, the anticipation for happiness in your life and the owning of your courage to conquer, will all trigger continual goodness. Try it; you'll see. Inspire and be inspired.

What it looks like to embrace your inner warrior

Remind yourself, you and only you can make choices for yourself. You are the only one that can make it or break it for yourself. Own it.

Positive thoughts bring positive energy. The power of manifestation, prayer and faith is real. Don't focus on what you don't want to happen; focus on what you do want to happen.

Face your emotions head-on. Acknowledge that they exist, and work through them as much as you can.

Advocate for yourself.

Find your passion and escape.

Follow your gut.

Kick fear to the curb and come to accept that fear is just a *mentality*, not a way of life.

Think: there's nothing wrong with you. You are not alone.

Detox your social circles.

Set boundaries.

Lead by example.

Don't be afraid to meet new people or join a club or a group; doing this opens so many doors.

Seek help, whether this means finding a new doctor(s), guidance counselor, therapist, a yoga class, a mindful retreat, a weekend road trip, reiki or a sabbatical to travel the world! Pick one or do it all!

Realize how precious and what a gift your health is, so do what you can to nurture it. Get yourself checked regularly. Be diligent.

Research, research, research. Never stop learning.

Be grateful for what you have, and fight for what you don't.

Everyone has their own story. Tell it proudly.

Be proud of what you've done for yourself and celebrate every positive step.

Don't judge others — this would imply there is a "norm" to judge by. And there simply isn't. Who says?

Jealousy is a waste of your time. Rise up and give others something to be jealous about, if they so choose to be.

We live in a society of endless pressures, where we're programmed to live our lives according to the expectations of others. Are our insecurities so substantial that we just give in to other people's opinions and views so easily that we sacrifice our own identity and what makes our *own* heart beat? Leave the what-ifs behind and take your leap. Whatever you may be going through, seek what you're looking for, however that looks for you. Everyone's experiences are unique. Whichever path you choose, I wholeheartedly hope you find your inner happiness and fulfillment.

Never let someone else dictate the fate of your own body. You know what you're feeling. Dissolve the doubts and go full speed ahead. Endometriosis is real, depression is real, cancer is real, helplessness is real; but don't just accept it as your reality. Make your <u>own</u> reality.

Ask yourself ...

Why not? (I mean truly ask yourself this.)
— If you are unable to come up with an actual legitimate answer, or you need some time to think about it, then you have no answer.

What is the absolute worst that can happen?
— Typically, you'll find with every answer that comes to mind, you will most likely discover a reasonable solution to that "worst" situation. Unless there is an unusual risk of death or a health risk, you can bounce back from anything else.

The first time I was challenged with this question was when I was contemplating whether I should apply to vet school. My then veterinarian coworker and now dear friend Dr. Collins asked me, as she held a dog spleen during surgery, "Why not?" I felt like a deer in headlights and could not seem to even pretend to have an answer to that question. I will never forget it. It was that moment that helped me to decide I would indeed pursue a career as a veterinarian. I just needed some help with a dose of reality. To this day, I thank Dr. Collins for that.

Challenge yourself and see what happens. What have you got to lose? After all, if most people are "comfort zoners" and followers, you can be a trendsetter. Find an outlet that works for you. We're creatures of habit and undoubtedly get caught in the day-to-day mundane, in the challenging web of parenthood, in the labyrinth of continual decisions, in the pressures of just about everything, you name it — until we find out we all have an inner beast just waiting to be discovered.

Set out to release your inner beast and make it contagious. Anything is possible.

Love yourself

Jackson & Stella
Rescues Rock!

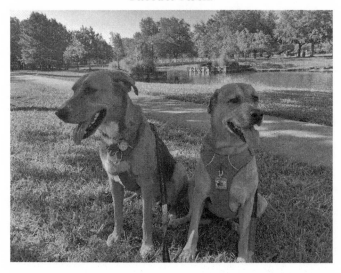

Made in the USA
Columbia, SC
03 December 2019